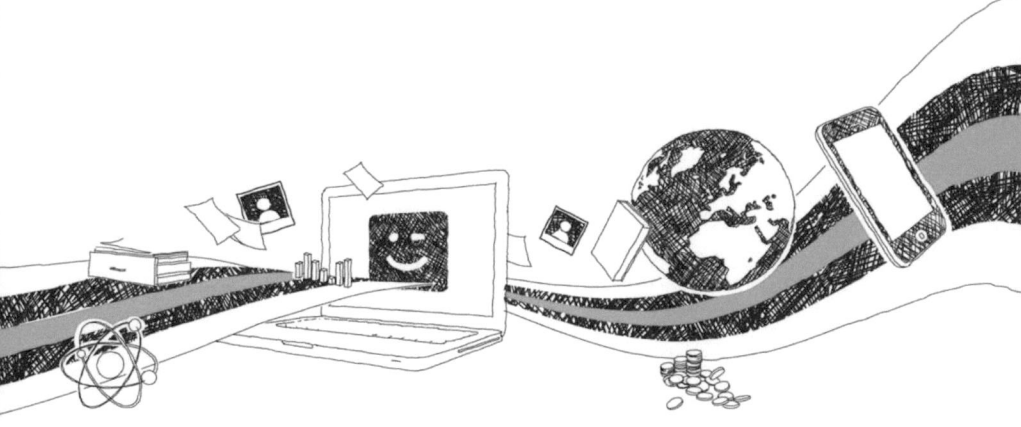
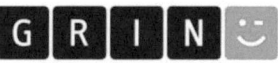

Christian Brugger

The essentials of Computed Tomography and its application in cardiac imaging

GRIN Publishing

Bibliographic information published by the German National Library:

The German National Library lists this publication in the National Bibliography; detailed bibliographic data are available on the Internet at http://dnb.dnb.de .

Imprint:

Copyright © 2011 GRIN Verlag GmbH
Print and binding: Books on Demand GmbH, Norderstedt Germany
ISBN: 978-3-640-97308-8

This book at GRIN:

http://www.grin.com/en/e-book/176173/the-essentials-of-computed-tomography-and-its-application-in-cardiac-imaging

GRIN - Your knowledge has value

Since its foundation in 1998, GRIN has specialized in publishing academic texts by students, college teachers and other academics as e-book and printed book. The website www.grin.com is an ideal platform for presenting term papers, final papers, scientific essays, dissertations and specialist books.

Technik
Informatik & Medien
Hochschule Ulm

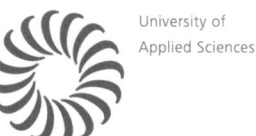

University of
Applied Sciences

THE ESSENTIALS OF COMPUTED TOMOGRAPHY AND ITS APPLICATION IN CARDIAC IMAGING

Medizinische Bildverarbeitung
(Medical image processing)
Information Systems (Master)
SS 2011

Christian Brugger B.Sc.

June 27th, 2011

Contents

Abstract

This paper introduces into the essentials of computed tomography and gives a brief lead-in to Cardiac CT, which is the clinical application of computed tomography in cardiac imaging. At first, the usage of X-rays is explained and the resulting main task of a CT scanner: The reconstruction of a three-dimensional image from the X-ray shadows, that are captured by the digital radiation detector unit. This reconstruction problem is known as the inverse problem in mathematics, which was initially solved by Johann Radon. Transferred to the field of computed tomography, the inverse problem means the definition of a volume dataset by reconstruction algorithms like for instance the Fourier Transform, which is shortly introduced, as well as the filtered backprojection. The main issue of Cardiac CT is the steady movement of the heart and chest of an examined patient. To ensure high image quality the scanner is triggered by a concurrently recorded ECG. ECG Triggering can ensure that the scanner only captues images during the phases of the heartbeat, where movement is minimal. One major application of Cardiac CT is non-invasive coronary angiography, which possibly could substitute invasive diagnostic surgeries like cardiac catheterization of non-emergency patients.

1

Introduction

In 1895, Wilhelm Conrad Röntgen invented a new type of radiation, which enabled physicians to visualize the inner structure of the human body. Starting with this first approach to produce diagnostic images in medicine, scientists have been steadily working on the improvement of imaging technologies based on the so called *X-rays*. A computer tomograph produces X-ray images, from every position around the patient's body. These recorded overlaying *shadows*, or *projections* from different angles have to be transformed into a slice, to get an image, that is interpretable by human beings.

In mathematics, this kind of reconstruction process is known as the *inverse problem*, which was primarily solved by Johann Radon in 1917. By capturing and computing many of these slices, a three dimensional model of the underlying body can be created, which provides a detailed view into the inside of the scanned tissue. "The invention of the [first] CT scanner in the late 1960s"[BS06, P. 1] is credited to Godfrey Hounsfield, which used a reconstruction algorithm based on "the mathematical fundaments published by Johann Radon"[OFB+06, P. 1], as also modern computer tomographs do today. The first working tomograph, "that could image the brain"[OFB+06, P. 1] was constructed by Hounsfield in 1971. One crucial difference between computed tomography by former scanners and modern ones is the time that the scanner needs to provide an 3D image of certain parts of the body. In the early ages of computed tomography, namely "during the 1960s and 1970s"[Buz08, P. 1], scanning one single slice took several minutes, what also resulted in a very huge amount of radiation, the patient was exposed to. Nowadays, one of the main goals is, to keep the radiation exposure as low as possible, which can be achieved by a scan time around milliseconds. Besides the general technical improvement of CT scanners, further applications of computed tomography have evolved. For instance the "introduction of the electron beam technology concept"[Sch04, P. 3], which was invented by Douglas Boyd in 1980 "moved CT into the realm of cardiac imaging."[Sch04, P. 3]

In the past computed tomography was the first and only "method to non-invasively acquire images of the inside of the human body."[Buz08, P. 1] Today it has become the main diagnostic technology in modern shock rooms, where it is used to get a fast overview of all injuries, an emergency trauma patient has suffered. But not only in case of emergency, computer tomographs are the first choice, also in cases where magnetic resonance imaging is not applicable, because for example the "object to be examined is dehydrated."[Buz08, P. 2]

2

Computed Tomography

2.1. X-rays (Roentgen rays)

Computer tomographs work with X-rays, that are produced by an X-ray generator, or X-ray tube. In this generator, electrons are accelerated from a cathode by high voltage. The electrons travel through a vacuum and are decelerated very fast by hitting a rotating anode disc, whereby different kinds of radioation are emitted, including X-rays. Through a small opening, the radiation is sent out directed towards the patient. After crossing the body, the X-rays encounter a detector, which is located at the opposite side.

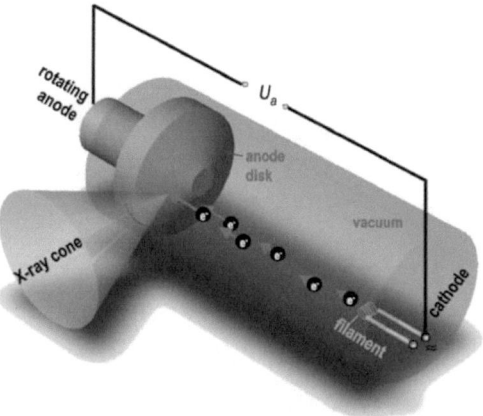

Figure 2.1.: Schematic drawing of an X-ray tube. [Buz08, Fig. 2.1.]

One crucial reason "for the wide exploitation of Röntgen's radiation"[Buz08, P. 15] was, that the generation as well as the detection of X-rays is very easy and can be achieved by quite "simple equipment."[Buz08, P. 15]

2.2. Inverse Problem

The tissues, which the X-rays go through, attenuate a certain amount of radiation, depending on their physical density. Bone structure for instance has a high density, so it appears in white or light grey, because the radiation is absorbed for the most part and only a marginal amount obtains the detector. Contrary to lungs that are full of air, which is visualized in dark grey or black. The amount of attenuation is measured in Hounsfield units (HU) typically at a range from -1000 to 5000. Consequently, to every type of tissue, a certain HU value can be determined, as listed in the *Hounsfield Scala* that is shown in figure 2.2.

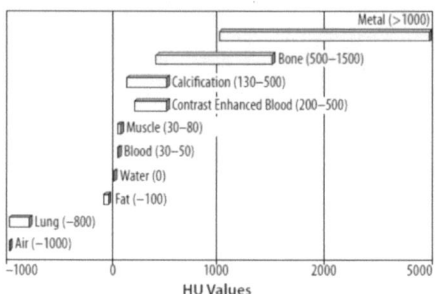

Figure 2.2.: Typical attenuation values of body structures and other objects, measured in Hounsfield units (HUs). [OFB⁺06, Fig. 1.4.]

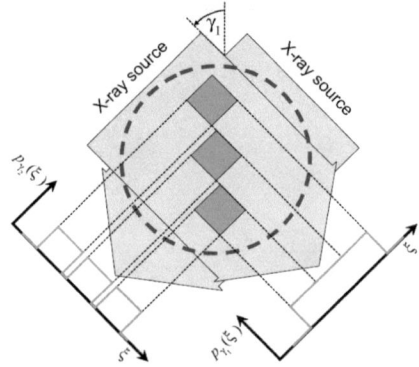

Figure 2.3.: Schematic illustration of computed tomography. [Buz08, Fig. 1.1.]

The CT scanner rotates around the patient to capture attenuation profiles from every perspective, or angle. Due to the fact that X-rays that cross a human body will of course successively cross many different types of tissue, the projection captured from one single perspective shows the summation of all the HU values of these tissues. The image, that is captured after one complete rotation shows the aggregated overlaying shadows of the scanned body, which leads to the "fundamental problem of computed tomography [...]: [The] Reconstruct[ion of] an object from its shadows or, more precisely, from its projections"[Buz08, P. 2], which is formally known as the inverse problem in mathematics.

In the domain of CT this means, to reproduce the three dimensional slice of the body from the overlaying two dimensional X-ray shadows, like illustrated in figure 2.4. Contrary to conventional X-ray examination, in computed tomography the radiation is not captured on a photosensitive film, which is developed afterwards, but rather converted into electrical impulses by a digital detector unit. These impulses are collected and translated into a slice image by a computer. After each complete rotation the patient table is moved ahead, so that the scanner is able to take the next slice. The aggregate of all recorded slices is then computed into a volume dataset, which finally can be visualized three-dimensionally. In modern, so called spiral CTs, this table movement is continuous, so that the scanner does not capture single slices but one proceeding helical image, from which the three-dimensional volume dataset is calculated directly.

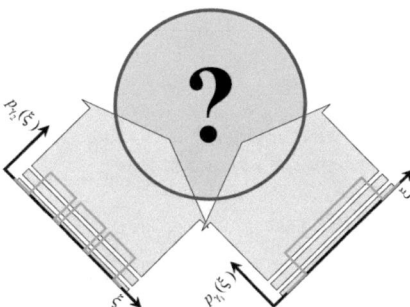

Figure 2.4.: Schematic illustration of the inverse problem. [Buz08, Fig. 1.2.]

3

Image Processing

3.1. Radon Transform

What the CT scanner mathematically does is, to produce line integrals from one layer of the scanned object over the attenuation coefficient μ. This line integral can be expressed as (cf. [Kas07, Slide 10]):

$$P = ln(\frac{I_0}{I}) = \int_s \mu ds$$

The summation of the integrals, captured from every perspective around the patient that lie on one plane, represents the projection of the irradiated slice, or its *Radon Transform*. After Radon, a function $f(x, y)$ is defined by the total of line integrals over this function (cf. [Leh04, Slide 15]):

$$\int_{-\infty}^{+\infty} f(x(l), y(l)) dl$$

The task of a computer tomograph is now the reconstruction of these projections, which is equivalent to the inversion of a Radon Transform. In practice, several methods can be used to achieve this goal. There are transformation procedures like the Fourier Transform, or algebraic methods like the direct matrix inversion, or iterative algorithms which approximate the reconstruction.

3.2. Fourier Transform

As one of the most important procedures for the inversion of the Radon Transform, at this point the *Fourier Transform* is briefly introduced. The Fourier Transform is a method to decompose a signal into a continious spectrum. In case of existence, it is defined as follows (cf. [Buz08, P. 118]),

$$F(u) = (\frac{\alpha}{2\pi})^{\frac{1}{2}} \int_{-\infty}^{+\infty} f(x) e^{-i\alpha ux} dx \equiv \mathcal{F}(f(x))$$

"where α is a constant whose origin is different in the field of signal processing from that in other applications."[Buz08, P. 118]

To obtain $f(x)$ from $F(u)$, the inverse of the Fourier Transform is used:

$$f(x) = (\frac{\alpha}{2\pi})^{\frac{1}{2}} \int\limits_{-\infty}^{+\infty} F(u)e^{i\alpha ux} du \equiv \mathcal{F}^{-1}(F(u))$$

In general, "with $f(x_1, x_2, x_3, \ldots, x_n)$ being a function of the n variables $x_1, x_2, x_3, \ldots, x_n$"[Buz08, P. 118], it can be expressed as:

$$F(u_1, \ldots, u_n) = (\frac{\alpha}{2\pi})^{\frac{1}{2}n} \int\limits_{-\infty}^{+\infty} \ldots \int\limits_{-\infty}^{+\infty} f(x_1, \ldots, x_n)e^{-i\alpha(u_1x_1 + \cdots + u_nx_n)} dx_1 \ldots dx_n$$

Which leads to its inverse:

$$f(x_1, \ldots, x_n) = (\frac{\alpha}{2\pi})^{\frac{1}{2}n} \int\limits_{-\infty}^{+\infty} \ldots \int\limits_{-\infty}^{+\infty} F(u_1, \ldots, u_n)e^{i\alpha(u_1x_1 + \cdots + u_nx_n)} du_1 \ldots du_n$$

3.3. Filtered backprojection

Another way to reconstruct a scanned slice from its captured projections is the *filtered backprojection*. As already mentioned, the projections represent the summation of all HU values of the tissues that the X-ray has crossed. In other words, the line integrals of the Radon Transform contain the sum of all pixels to reconstruct, but there is no information on the corresponding position. The approach of this method is, to evenly contribute the value of the integral to the original integration way. By repeatedly overlaying all projection lines in every point (x, y) of the slice image, it reconstructed aproximately.

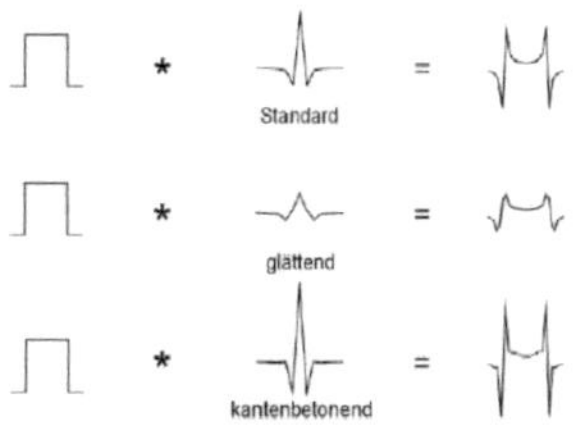

Figure 3.1.: Convolution kernels used for filtered backprojection: Standard, smoothing, edge emphasizing. [Leh04, Slide 43]

The major issue of backprojection is, that it leads to blurring. To minimize this problem, the original profile is multiplied with a suitable convolution kernel, to achieve a filtered profile that then can be used for backprojection. Three of those filters are shown in figure 3.1. The influence of these convolution kernels can be seen in figure 3.2

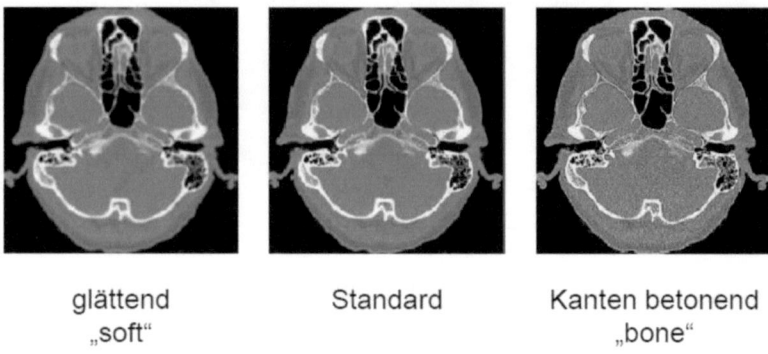

| glättend | Standard | Kanten betonend |
| „soft" | | „bone" |

Figure 3.2.: The influence of filtering with convolution kernels: Smoothing, standard, edge emphasizing. [Leh04, Slide 46]

4

Cardiac CT

A relatively new application, regarding the long history of computed tomography, is *Cardiac CT*. This non-invasive technique to acquire diagnostic images of the human heart is not completely established in clinical practice yet, but has possibly the capability to substitute invasive diagnostic methods, such as cardiac catheterization, in cases where no percutaneous coronary intervention (PCI) is needed immediately. Additionally there are indications, where Cardiac CT is the method of choice, for instance the "triage of patients with stable angina"[OFB+06, P. 188] for planning purpose of non-invasive treatment, or the "follow-up investigation after stent placement"[OFB+06, P. 188] within a PCI surgery.

4.1. ECG Triggering

In consequence of its steady movement, taking pictures of the heart with any diagnostic imaging device is problematic. Therefore, "motion artifacts can significantly affect cardiovascular CT images"[BS06, P. 19], which can be caused by the heartbeat itself or by breathing movement of the chest. Modern scanners working with "multidetector CT and electron beam CT techniques"[BS06, p. 19] provide the possibility to complete a scan within one single breath-hold, which minimizes the artifacts from respiration, but since the motion of the cardiac muscle is very complex and not directly controllable, the computer tomograph has to capture the images "preferably in the diastolic phase, when cardiac motion is minimal"[OFB+06, P. 76]. The very short scanning time can be reached by concurrent acquisition of multiple slices. Nowerdays computed tomography works with "up to 64 narrowly collimated slices."[BS06, P. 123]

By simultaniously recording an ECG, the scanner can be triggered to only acquire data within a defined time period during this phase of the cardiac cycle. Though, due to the fact that no ECG rhythm is exactly constant, especially not the one of patients, suffering from a heart condition, determining the optimal time window is difficult. In practice, there are three different approaches to select the trigger moment. "The best image quality can be obtained in mid-diastolic phase"[OFB+06, P. 107], or in other words, in the middle of the time interval between two R-waves, which is defined as $\delta_{RR} = 50\%$. Alternatively "the end-systolic phase"[OFB+06, P. 107] starting at $\delta_{RR} = 30\%$ was shown to be appropriate.

- The easiest approach is, to define a static *absolute delay* T_{del} from the the latest R-wave to approximately reach the optimal triggering moment. (See figure 4.1c)

- Another *prospective* strategy is, to determine the trigger by calculating a *relative delay* from the latest R-wave, dependent on the absolute R to R time span T_{RR} of the current cardiac cycle. (See figure 4.1a)

- Contrary to the first two methods, *retrospective* triggering can be used, where an *absolut reverse* T_{rev} to the next R-wave, which therefore is independent from T_{RR}, is calculated. (See figure 4.1b)

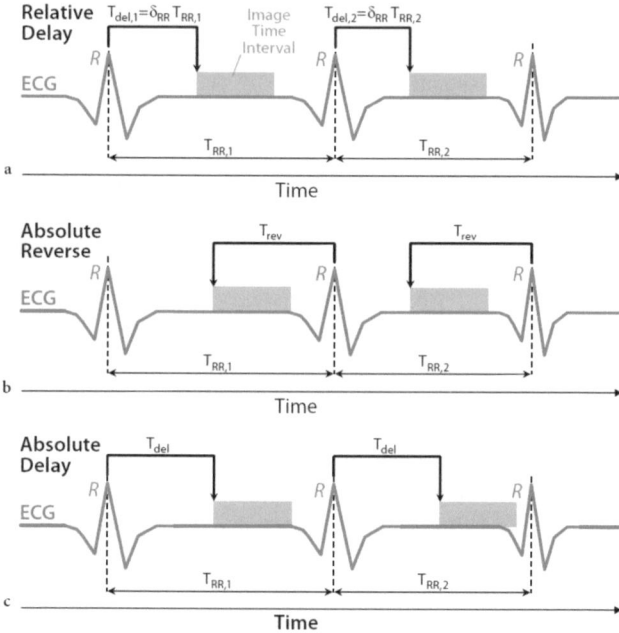

Figure 4.1.: Phase definition for ECG triggering and ECG gating by selection of the start point of the temporal data interval within every heart cycle. [OFB$^+$06, Fig. 4.34a-c]

In practice, when using retrospective ECG triggering, the scanner acquires data throughout the entire scan and afterwards the optimal time windows are evaluated for the image reconstruction. Which is one of the main differences to and the main advantage of prospective triggering, where the scanner does only irradiate the patient within the defined time windows, what leads to deutlicheTODO "limitation to radiation exposure."[BS08, P. 3] The crucial disadvantage is, that there is no guarantee, that the hereby selected time window is optimal, because there is no adjustion to sudden frequency changes. If the reconstructed images contain significant movement artifacts, in the worst case, the entire scan has to be repeated.

4.2. Coronary CT Angiography

As explained before, one major application of Cardiac CT in clinical practice is the non-invasive coronary angiography for diagnostic purpose in patients with coronary heart disease or as a follow-up investigation after PCI surgeries. The task of a coronary angiograpy examination is to achieve high resolution images of the small arteries surrounding the heart, which supply the myocardium with oxygenated blood, in order to detect stenoses or even closures that cause cardiac infarction. The other way round, lesions of the coronary vessels or constrictions can be excluded for differencial diagnosis of chest pain.

For imaging the coronary vessels, which typically have a small lumen of "1 to 4mm"[BS06, P. 123], usually the injection of contrast media is necessary, which "raises the density in the blood pool well above that of the vessel wall and surrounding tissue."[BS06, P. 123] As previously mentioned, the attenuation profiles captured by the scanner project the physical densities of the crossed tissues, so consequently on the resulting image, the contrast between blood and vessel is higher, which allows an easier optical distinction.

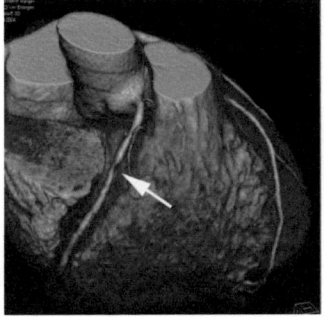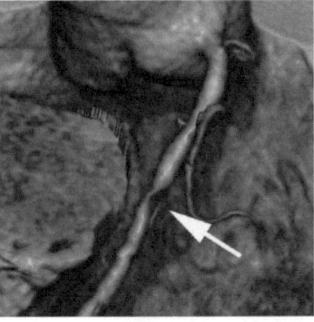

Figure 4.2.: Stenosis of the right coronary artery in a 3D volume-rendered reconstruction. [BS06, Fig. 9.6]

Bibliography

[BS06]   Matthew J. Budoff and Jerold S. Shinbane. *Cardiac CT Imaging: Diagnosis of Cardiovascular Disease.* Springer, 2006.

[BS08]   Matthew J. Budoff and Jerold S. Shinbane. *Handbook of Cardiovascular CT: Essentials for Clinical Practice.* Springer, 2008.

[Buz08]   Thorsten M. Buzug. *Computed Tomography: From Photon Statistics to Modern Cone-Beam CT.* Springer, 2008.

[Kas07]   Stefan Kasperl. *Grundlagen und Anwendungen industrieller Computertomographie.* 2007. [http://www.ndt.net/article/dgzfp07/Inhalt/v15.pdf; accessed 06/14/2011].

[Leh04]   Klaus Lehnertz. *Computer-Tomographie/Computed Tomography: Grundlagen/Basics.* 2004. [http://epileptologie-bonn.de/cms/upload/ homepage/lehnertz/CT1.pdf; accessed 06/14/2011].

[OFB⁺06] Bernd M. Ohnesorge, Thomas G. Flohr, Christoph R. Becker, Andreas Knez, and Maximilian F. Reiser. *Multi-slice and Dual-source CT in Cardiac Imaging: Principles - Protocols - Indications - Outlook.* Springer, 2006.

[PLLP06] Guillem Pons-Lladó and Rubén Leta-Petracca. *Atlas of Non-Invasive Coronary Angiography by Multidetector Computed Tomography (Developments in Cardiovascular Medicine).* Springer, 2006.

[Sch04]   U. Joseph Schoepf. *CT of the Heart: Principles and Applications.* Humana Press, 2004.

List of Figures